Come Breathe With Us

For the Health of It

Trudy Baker

A series of self-healing techniques, breathing patterns, rhythms and exercises that foster optimum health

ISBN-13:
978-0991684847

ISBN-10:
0991684842

DEDICATION

To all my healing friends, energy healers, light-workers, and alternative healing practitioners. To those of you I personally know as my teachers and students. To those of you whose webinars I have attended, whose books I have read. I have learned from you all. To all people who work for the promotion of alternative non-invasive and drug-free healing for the planet and all who live on it.

.

CONTENTS

ACKNOWLEDGMENTS

Thanks to Miriam Orta, Yuri Orta and Claire Morrisseau for being part of the first run of the Come Breathe With Us workshop. Your participation and your input has been extremely valuable. A special thumbs up for Miriam Orta for all her efforts and time spent to support, and promote fine-tuning the second run of the workshop in Laredo. Many thanks to Diane Michaud for the anatomical background information. Above all I am much appreciative of my husband Everett's editorial expertise, support and patience with me for all the time it kept me at my desk.

PREFACE

The techniques and methods presented are not original to IEHealers. They are a combination of teachings of ancient and more modern healing modalities compiled by Trudy and Everett Baker.

 It is our willingness to share our time and talents for the highest good of the people we meet to promote self-healing the natural way.

Our approach is Intermodal. Although we are trained in many modalities, we do not favor any one over another. We have experienced the ease and seamlessness with which several healing modalities integrate with each other, and wish to promote self-healing.

Material may be reproduced for personal reference material or as an aid for the teaching of energy healing techniques by the Team Members of our sister organization ShifaHouse International or by permission from IEHealers.

INTRODUCTION TO BREATHING

Why Breathing?

Many if not most energy healing modalities place a lot of emphasis on breathing techniques. Some critics are of the opinion that a healing modality which does not place a lot of emphasis on breathing cannot be very effective.

Think of the many every day expressions and idioms that refer to breathing as key to our very being. Here are some. *The breath of life. *Take a deep breath. *Don't breathe a word of it. * Breathe a sigh of relief. *Breathe down someone's neck. *Don't have time to take a breath. *Breathe one's last. *Being out of breath.

Do you want to get rid of stress, anxiety, insomnia, depression or memory loss? Have you been tired all the time lately? Improved breathing will help you restore the oxygen level in all your organs, and cells. You will regain your brain health, your vitality and overall health.

In this booklet I will show you to breathe effectively to improve your everyday health. Taking the on-line course or the life workshop will help you to build up resistance against diseases like Pneumonia, Asthma, Bronchitis and Cystic Fibrosis, common diseases of the respiratory system.

You will learn to become aware of your own breathing patterns. You'll discover whether you normally do chest breathing or abdominal breathing. Some diseases associated with poor breathing habits can be avoided and healed by effective breathing. You will learn how to clear a stuffy nose without medication. Practicing various breathing rhythms will help you find the most efficient rhythm for your daily health. Double nostril breathing and Mentalphysics breathing exercises will soon become part of your daily breathing routine to maintain good health.

When I read the story of Laura Applegren, I became convinced that I needed to learn what she learned and share that knowledge with all my friends, and with many more.

The Story of Laura Applegren

Come to the desert and learn to breathe.

When Pranic Healing teacher, Master Stephen Co, went to teach a workshop in Chicago around the year 2000 a 92 year old woman enrolled in his class. He was told by the event organizers who knew her that she would easily be able to keep up with the rigorous routine of the workshop. She was known to walk around the block at a pace that most 30 something year olds could not keep up with. Her name was Laura Applegren. Here's her story.

Laura was diagnosed with breast cancer in her early 40's. Her doctors in Wisconsin, where she lived, wanted to do a mastectomy immediately. She declined. She read an advert in a magazine: "Knowledge is Power. Come to the desert and learn to breathe". It was an advert by the Institute of Mentalphysics. Against her husband's wishes she went for a week to learn to breathe with Edwin J. Dingle. After doing the exercises for a while her cancer completely disappeared. She lived for 50 more years. She led the breathing exercises in Stephen Co's class and the students much younger than Laura were amazed at her vitality. When she died a few years later in her sleep she still had all her natural teeth, had never needed glasses, nor hearing aids.

BREATHING PATTERNS

Which way do you breathe?

All of us are breathing. Breathing amplifies the life force. Most alternative healing modalities require FULL breathing practices.

Many of us are used to shallow breathing. Shallow breathers use the upper chest, or shoulders. Practicing a new breathing technique may feel uncomfortable to start with but with a little practice you'll soon do it without even thinking about it.

I read an article on line at www.morethanmedication.ca titled Bad breath, good breath. "As automatic as it is, many people may not be breathing very well. Tension, poor posture or ill-fitting clothing cause many of us to take very shallow breaths."

You can tell when you're breathing shallowly if you can see or feel your ribcage moving out as you inhale. You may even be taking in so little air that your chest barely moves at all. If that's the case, then you're breathing with the muscles in between your ribs instead of with your diaphragm, the powerful muscle at the bottom of your chest cavity that pulls air down."

How many times have you heard the expressions "take a deep breath" and "breathe through your diaphragm"?

If you're not really sure how to breathe through your diaphragm, try this exercise.

Bring out your yoga mat.

Start by lying on the floor on your back. It will make it easier to develop the proper deep breathing technique.
Place one hand on your upper chest and the other on your belly just above your waist.
Breathe in slowly through your nose. You should feel the hand on your belly rise.
Breathe out slowly through your mouth. The hand on your belly should gradually lower.
Repeat a few times, then focus on allowing your
ribcage to expand and widen as your belly. moves out, so that you are filling up your entire lungs, from bottom to top.

- ✓ **Focused breathing is key to your ability to facilitate healing.**
- ✓ **Most alternate healing modalities emphasize focused breathing techniques.**
- ✓ **Shallow breathers use the upper chest or the shoulders.**
- ✓ **Full breathing engages the diaphragm.**

Regular practice of the exercises combined with the breathing patterns as explained on these pages has specific physical benefits, including but not limited to

- ✓ it brings more oxygen into the body
- ✓ it wakes up the whole body and makes it more responsive

- ✓ it releases muscles of upper body, scapula (shoulder blade), sternum (breast bone) and ribs, allowing for better rotation of upper body
- ✓ it releases tension in the torso: opening up the ribcage and diaphragm. releasing tension in the trunk where it connects to the lumbar plexus
- ✓ it opens up the energy flow in pelvis, sacrum, tailbone
- ✓ it releases tension and increases flexibility in the muscles of the pelvis
- ✓ it forces cleansing of the air passages cleaning and energizing the head and the spinal column all the way down to the tailbone
- ✓ it prevents, minimizes and corrects the need for adult diapers
- ✓ it helps maintain one's sense of balance

How much will you actually benefit from the exercises? It will vary depending on your health, your condition and your commitment to doing the work. Here's a story of what it did for one person.

Hi, I am Susana Morton

I attended the "Come Breathe With Us" workshop taught by Trudy Baker, in Laredo Texas in July 2015. All my life I have suffered from allergies and respiratory problems. Three years ago I got sick with bronchitis and I was diagnosed with asthma. Since then I have to take medications every day. I also use a nebulizer everyday with more medication up to 4 times a day.

I always got episodes of lack of air and my throat would be closed. I had frequent coughing spells when I was sleeping up to 3 or 4 times a night, and often in the day time. I could be anywhere: at the bank, at the store, watching TV, in family reunions, with friends. I took the Mentalphysic breathing Workshop for my health. To my surprise by the 2nd day of the workshop I noticed that when I coughed I was not lacking air and I could control the cough. On the 3rd day of the workshop I stopped using the nebulizer by my own decision because I started feeling a lot better and so well that I even forget to use it. And even the medication for my sinus issues, I stopped using them completely because now I can breathe perfectly. I do my mentalphysic breathing throughout the day. I do them again before I go to sleep.

Various types of breathing

The diaphragm is the most efficient muscle for breathing. It is a large, dome-shaped muscle located at the base of the lungs. Your abdominal muscles help move the diaphragm and give you more power to empty your lungs.

Chronic obstructive pulmonary disease (COPD) may prevent the diaphragm from working effectively. When you have pulmonary disease, air often becomes trapped in the lungs, pushing down on the diaphragm. The neck and chest muscles must then assume an increased share of the work of breathing. This can leave the diaphragm weakened and flattened, causing it to work less efficiently.

Clavicular breathing
Fills the top third of your lungs
> A very shallow type of breathing
> Employs the raising of collar bones and shoulders
> Used by most overweight persons
> Used by many smokers
> Frequently (temporarily) adopted by pregnant women

Intercostal breathing
Fills up the top and middle parts of the lungs
> Employs the pulling up of shoulders and expanding the rib cage
> Employs the muscles around the chest; it is hard work
> Commonly employed by athletes during competitions

Diaphragmatic breathing or abdominal breathing or sometimes known as "belly breathing"
Fills up the entire lungs
> Uses the abdominal muscles which engages the diaphragm
> A greater amount of air is brought into the lungs

It provides more energetic benefits

Practice Diaphragmatic Breathing

When you first learn the diaphragmatic breathing technique, it may be easier for you to follow the instructions lying down, as shown. As you gain more practice, you can try the diaphragmatic breathing technique while sitting in a chair as shown on the next page.

Lie flat on your back on a level surface. Support your head with a pillow and your knees as well. Rest one hand lightly on your upper chest and the other just below your rib cage on your stomach. It allows you to feel your diaphragm move as you breathe.

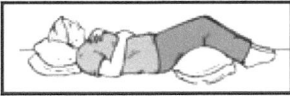

Breathe in slowly through your nose so that your stomach moves out against your hand. The hand on your chest remains as still as possible.

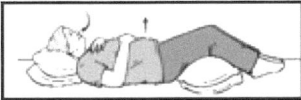

As you exhale through pursed lips, pull in and tighten your stomach muscles, collapsing them inward. The hand on your chest remains as still as possible.

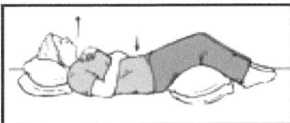

Try again if at first you don't succeed.

Diaphragmatic Breathing in a Chair

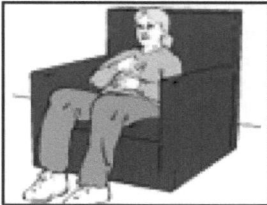

Sit comfortably, with your knees bent and your shoulders, head and neck relaxed. Rest one hand lightly on your upper chest and the other just below your rib cage on your stomach. It allows way you to feel your diaphragm move as you breathe.

Breathe in slowly through your nose so that your stomach moves out against your hand. The hand on your chest remains as still as possible.

As you exhale through pursed lips, pull in and tighten your stomach muscles, collapsing them inward. The hand on your chest remains as still as possible.

Try again if at first you did not succeed.

One of the advantage of abdominal breathing is *that it assists with lymphatic drainage. The lymphatic system is effectively the body's sewerage system, draining away waste materials and excess fluid. As the lymphatic system does not have a heart to pump the waste throughout the body, it is reliant on the motions of the muscles, including the diaphragm. During abdominal breathing, lymph is sucked through the bloodstream, neutralizing and destroying dead cells, reducing fluid retention, and improving detoxification of the body. By utilizing the natural benefits of abdominal breathing you will improve the quality of your blood flow, increase delivery of oxygen to working muscles, and reduce the symptoms of anxiety associated with over-breathing.*

McKeown, Patrick. The Oxygen Advantage: The Simple, Scientifically Proven Breathing Techniques for a Healthier, Slimmer, Faster, and Fitter Life

Traditional Chinese Taoism advocates Abdominal Breathing

The traditional Chinese philosophy of Taoism succinctly describes ideal breathing as "so smooth that the fine hairs within the nostrils remain motionless." True health and inner peace occurs when breathing is quiet, effortless, soft, through the nose, abdominal, rhythmic, and gently paused on the exhale. This is how human beings naturally breathed until modern life changed everything.

IMPEDIMENTS TO BREATHING

Negative Postural Conditioning often is the cause of poor breathing habits. As children we are taught to stand tall and straight. Military training teaches "Chest out, stomach in!" Fitness images glorify flat stomach and straight back.

Holding negative emotions is another reason many of us breathe poorly. When afraid one is scared to breathe. When angry one holds one's breath, and stress creates tension in the diaphragm.

Chronic over-breathing is another common cause of poor health. Many people take in two or three time more oxygen than they need without knowing it. Taking in too much air on a regular basis causes breathlessness when doing exercises or physical work.

Lack of awareness also is a common cause of shallow breathing. We've been conditioned to shallow breathing. Many of us simply do not know we could be healthier if we breathed more effectively.

Some diseases are associated with poor breathing

Pneumonia, Asthma, Bronchitis and Cystic Fibrosis are common diseases of the respiratory system. One of the main contributing factors causing these diseases is poor breathing habits. Poor breathing weakens the cells of the lungs and the airways, making them vulnerable to attack of viruses and pathogens.

The good news is that many of the diseases mentioned can be reversed by good breathing habits, without drugs and without surgery.

To reduce the negative effects of poor breathing you can practice slow, gentle, relaxed, calm, and quiet breathing through the nose and engaging the diaphragm.

Read on, and learn to breathe for improved health.

EASY TO LEARN EVERY DAY EXERCISES

Clearing a Stuffy Nose

Over 85% of people can make their stuffy nose clear in less than 1 minute if they follow instructions correctly. The remedy was tested on more than 100,000 people. This simple breathing exercise of how to clear a stuffy nose or get rid of nasal congestion was developed by Russian doctors practicing the Buteyko breathing method.

These Nose Clearing Tips are for people just with a stuffy nose, not for chronic sinus problems or nasal polyps.

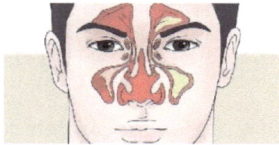

1. Sit back relaxed in an upright position on a dining room chair.
2. Breath out, through your nose or mouth.
3. Keep your mouth shut during the rest of the exercise for optimum results.
4. Hold your breath by pinching your nose shut.
5. Gently nod your head, up and down.
6. Hold until the first minimal level of discomfort.
7. Breathe in through the nose (make an effort to keep your mouth shut.)

At this point the stuffy nose is cleared and you can keep breathing comfortably through your nose.

BRON WROTE ME THE FOLLOWING NOTE:

"ME AND MY KIDS TRIED THIS. IT REALLY DOES WORK."

The above exercise does more than clear a stuffy nose. Daily consecutive repetitions of the exercise with 30 to 60 seconds breaks between rounds, over an extended period of time will increase your ability to hold your breath. The longer you can hold your breath, the less likely you will become short of breath while doing exercise. The "hold" periods in between breaths improve the blood's capacity to transport oxygen through the body. People with respiratory diseases such as asthma will gain greatly by doing the exercise. They will not only feel better, but also the asthma will greatly reduce in severity, with fewer and fewer attacks further apart.

Falling Asleep in 60 seconds

For a long time, I had a hard time sleeping. We can chalk it up to bad food late at night, too many screens before bed, and stress. I found it incredibly difficult to shut my brain down and give it a break at night. After weeks of not being able to sleep a full night, a friend of mine told me about the "4-7-8" breathing technique.

This method was developed by a wellness practitioner, Harvard-educated Dr. Andrew Weil, who studies meditation and breathing, and how it can be used to counteract stress. It's easy to do. It involves regulating your breathing to various counts of 4, 7 and 8. It lets oxygen better fill the lungs, calms the mind and relaxes muscles.

You breathe in through your nose for four seconds, hold it for seven seconds, and exhale through your mouth for eight seconds. It slows down your heart rate and it also releases chemicals in your brains that soothe you.

1. Lie on your back on your bed and relax.
2. Breathe in through your nose for 4 seconds.
3. Hold for 7 seconds.
4. Breathe out for 8 seconds.
5. Repeat for several times.

After 60 seconds you will likely be asleep. Try again if at first you did not succeed.

Why We Yawn

When learning the Metalphysic breathing exercises I found myself yawning more frequently than usual, and began to wonder about it. I had always thought that one yawns when bored or tired. Certainly, I was not bored when learning the new breathing routines, nor tired. An hour of focused breathing invigorates me. It did when I started learning the exercises; it still does now when my husband and I regularly practice the Mentalphysic exercises. During the "Come Breathe With Us" workshops, I noticed the students also began to yawn. Did I bore them that much? Were they so tired?

Again, I wondered and began to do some research. I like to share some of the things I learned other people say about why we yawn.

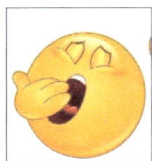

A dictionary definition of yawning is: "involuntarily opening one's mouth wide and inhaling deeply due to tiredness or boredom." There is more to it, though, I believe. Most people have experienced that yawning appears to be contagious. Several sources I read state that it is a copycat behavior which could improve one's alertness. Good hint. Next time I am teaching I will start to yawn and in such a way encourage my audience to greater alertness. ☺ I may even experiment with putting a picture of a yawn on every page I write to start my readers yawning, allowing them to read and absorb the material with greater alertness and ease.

Studies about why people yawn have a long history. According to the ancient philosopher Hippocrates, we yawn to expel bad air that has accumulated in our bodies. Ahh, so yawning is an ancient healing technique. It's been shown that while yawning one uses the bottom parts of one's lungs, thus it removes stale air from the lungs which certainly is good for one's health. But since we start yawning unconsciously and spontaneously and cannot do so on command we depend on our subconscious brain to use it as a healing method. A good yawn apparently cools the brain as well and hence makes the brain function more effectively.

Many articles I read agree that yawning is a way to help our body and mind transition from one behavioral state to another, such as from sleep to wakefulness and vice versa, from anxiety to calm, and from boredom to alertness.

According to Michael Decker, Ph.D., associate professor at the Frances Payne Bolton School of Nursing at the Western Reserve University and a spokesperson for the American Academy of Sleep Medicine, yawning is a self-correcting mechanism to shallow breathing. He goes on to explain that an open-mouthed yawn causes the sinus walls "to expand and contract like a bellows" pumping air into our brain which lowers the brain temperature. Therefore, when learning new stuff at a rapid rate we need to cool our brain to lower the temperature to remain alert.

I always feel a smile coming onto my face when my students in a workshop begin to yawn. To me it means that changes are starting to happen at a subconscious level.

The Movements

The Mentalphysic exercises combine breathing and retention rhythms with gentle physical exercises. The exercises are not strenuous and care needs to be taken to not stretch, bob and bend beyond a level that is anatomically comfortable. The movements build on each other and it is advisable to follow the order shown. For people who have particular physical challenges it is important not to overdo a certain stretch or bend. We repeatedly mention the line, "as far as you comfortably can". If you can not do a certain movement, you can do it in your imagination, still combining the breathing rhythm with the imaginary movements. Many of the sources I have read maintain that the subconscious mind does not know the difference between real and imaginary. There is great benefit in doing imaginary exercises.

BREATHING RHYTHMS

Pay attention to your own breathing a moment. Count the number of seconds you inhale and how many seconds you exhale. Do you inhale for the same count as exhale?

Now take a deep breath. Did you inhale, or did you exhale first? Which took longer?

In the chart below are a number of basic breathing rhythms. Notice that both the 1- 4 and 2 - 6 breaths proportionately take more time breathing out than breathing in. This emphasizes the importance to completely empty the lungs. When the lungs are empty, one breathes in automatically. Some yogi breathing techniques support this idea in teaching to lead with the out breath.

I recommend you practice each rhythm for 5 or 6 times adjusting to normal breathing in between each set of breaths. Do this once in the morning and again in the evening. During the course of the day stop a moment now and then and pay attention what breathing rhythm you are using when not focusing on it. After a week or so of regular practice of the different rhythms you will find which rhythm is best for you.

- **the 4 - 4 breath;** in to the count of 4, out to the count of 4

- **the 2 - 4 breath;** in to the count of 2, out to the count of 4

- **the 6 - 3 - 6 - 3** breath; in to the count of 6 , hold 3, out to the count of 6, hold 3

- **the 6 - 6 – 3 breath; in to the count of 6, out to the count of 6, hold 3**

The 7 -1 - 7 – 1 Breath

This is an advanced Pranic breathing technique used to completely empty the lungs of stale air. It is known in the Jewish tradition as Kosher Yoga. Also known in Pranic Healing as an Optimum Breathing Rhythm.
The length of the counts is not as important as keeping a steady rhythm. A good pacing technique is to use one's pulse count. timing breathing and retention to one's pulse. As one progresses, the pulse count will slow down.

1. Place your tongue on your palate and keep it there for the entire exercise.
2. Inhale for 7 counts.
3. Hold for 1 count.
4. Exhale for 7 counts.
5. Hold for 1 count.
6. Perform 3 sets of 10 cycles (#2 - #5 is one cycle) with one minute pause between sets.

WARM UPS TO MENTALPHYSIC EXERCISES

The warm up exercises are done sitting on a dining room chair with both feet flat on the floor and back erect. For the Bobble Head exercise inhale through the nose and exhale through the mouth. The rest of the exercises are done standing, feet slightly less than shoulder width apart. Knees straight but relaxed. In all the exercises inhale through the nose and exhale through the mouth.

Double Nostril Breathing

Also known as single nostril breathing or alternate nostril breathing and as the Harmonic Breath. Different modalities teach slightly varying methods of what basically is the same technique.

Most people while awake breathe through one nostril for about 90 minutes, then switch over through the other for about 90 minutes. During the switch over period, usually about 10 minutes we breathe through both nostrils. When breathing through the right nostril the left side of the brain is supplied with oxygen, and vice versa. During the switch over period both sides of the brain are supplied with oxygen. That's when both the intuitive and the analytical part of our brains work in unison, or coherently. That's when we have our "Aha!" moments. Not all of us have the same rhythm, some of us oxidize our right side of the brain for a slightly longer time than the left, and some the other way. I.E. some of us are more analytical and some more intuitive. It may also be the reason why most people toss from sleeping on one side to sleeping on the other side to maintain some sort of balance.

Before starting the exercise test if you take in breath equally through both nostrils by pinching one nostril and taking a few breaths. Then through the other. Most people will find that it is easier to breathe through one side than through the other. At the end of the exercise do this test again.

This exercise trains us to breathe through both nostrils simultaneously for longer periods of time, creating increased left / right brain coherence.

Double nostril breathing takes us into what is known as a Theta Brain Wave mode. Similar effect can be attained by deep meditation.

In Core Transformation this state is referred to as being in the Core Point. HeartMath refers to it as Point Zero.

The hand position are as follows

- Right thumb resting on right nostril
- Right ring finger resting on left nostril
- Index and middle finger pointing towards the middle of the forehead (third eye)

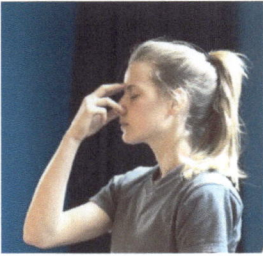

Try it:

a. Breathe out comfortably.
b. Hold your left nostril closed.
 Through the right nostril breathe in for 6,
 hold for 3,
 breathe out for 6,
 hold for 3.
c. Hold your right nostril closed.
 Through the left nostril breathe in for 6,
 hold for 3,
 breathe out for 6,
 hold for 3.
d. Repeat for a total of 7 cycles.

The Bobble Head

The Bobble head Breath is also known as the Rapid Turtle Breath.

The exercise is a forced cleansing of the air passages. It cleans and energizes the head and the spinal column all the way down to the tailbone. The vigorous head movements pull the energy up and down your spine.

The exercise benefits the neck muscles and the cervical spinal
nerves.

The Bobblehead Exercise

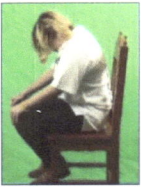

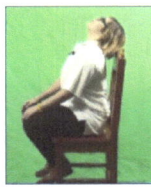

The second picture shows the head back as far as it should be for the Bobblehead exercise.
Move back and forth as far as you comfortably can, making sure not to over-do it at the beginning.

Here's the exercise:
* Tuck your chin against your chest.
* Inhale through the nose.
* Tilt *(bob)* your head as far back as it can comfortable go.
* Coordinate tilt and inhale so that your lungs are full when your head is back.
* Exhale through the mouth while bringing the chin back to the chest.
* Exhale forcibly and audibly with a *shu*, stay relaxed.

- Coordinate the head movement and exhale so that when your lungs are empty your chin is back on your chest.
- Do a set of 14 cycles (breaths/bobs).
- Take a break between each of the 14 sets of the 14 bobs.
- The last set only needs to be 7 bobs / head movements.
- If you feel dizzy take a longer break and walk around for a few minutes.

MENTALPHYSIC BREATHING EXERCISES

All the remaining exercises are done standing up, feet slightly less than shoulder width apart. Knees straight but relaxed. In all the exercises inhale through the nose and exhale through the mouth, unless specifically instructed otherwise. It is recommended to take a few normal breaths between the exercises and pay attention to how your body feels. Normal breathing is done through the nose, keeping the mouth shut. Walk around some between the different sets of exercises until your breathing normalizes.

Claire's Story

*At first the breathing exercises were quite challenging for me.
Holding my breath while moving the head or arms would give
me a headache. I had to do them all sitting down instead of
standing up.*

*Now at the end of the workshop I can do them all standing up,
at my own pace and making the holding time shorter.*

*I noticed that after a few days I could stand in the kitchen to
cook with almost no back pain. Usually standing for a long
time is very challenging for my back.*

*Trudy and Everett are very dedicated and patient teachers who
really care about their students.*

I immediately felt comfortable living with them.

*Besides the workshop on breathing techniques we did healing
circles where everyone participated in working for one of us.*

*One on one sessions using different modalities took place here
and there in an informal way.*

We all helped each other in a very loving atmosphere.

*All and all it's been a very healing and enriching experience
which I highly recommend to anyone who's willing to take
charge of their health and wellbeing.*

The Vital Breath

The vital Breath was originally known as the revitalizing breath. Although this exercise does not involve any movement of the arms, legs and trunk of the body, it energizes the whole body and improves overall responsiveness for all of all spinal nerves. **It wakes up and energizes the entire back**

Nerves of the spine:

Cervical spinal nerves, Atlas to C 7 (the neck)
Spinal accessory nerve, which is a cranial nerve controlling nerves from brain to neck and upper shoulder (SCM and Trapezius)
The thoracodorsal nerve (T 1 – 7)
The pectoral nerves (around the shoulders)
Intercostal nerves (thorax to abdominal wall)
The femoral nerve (from lower spine to upper leg bone)
The inferior gluteal nerve (L5 to S2) lower back to hips
The superior gluteal nerve (Solar plexus to sciatica) L4 and 5 to S 1

When doing the Vital Breath, keep your mouth nearly closed and teeth slightly touching. Keep feet and ankles together, or just short of shoulder width apart. Keep your spine and neck erect. Keep your fingers straight and together.

The Vital Breath Exercises

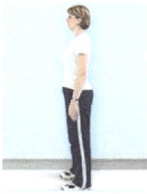

Stand in the position shown.

- Exhale audibly until lungs are empty. Snort to expel any and all remaining air from the lungs.
- Inhale deeply until lungs are full.
- Take a final sniff in through the nose to fill your lungs even more and hold.
- Tense your neck muscles, jaws, arms and legs, torso and buttocks, squeeze your PC muscles*.
- Hold your breath to the count of 5.
- Exhale audible through your teeth.
- When your lungs are empty, snort out all remaining air and hold to the count of 5.
- Relax all muscles.
- Take a few normal breaths.
- Pay attention to how your body feels

Alternatively, do this exercise to the count of 6 - 3 - 6 - 3

*The PC muscles, pubococcygeal muscles, run from the pubic area through the perineum (abdominal floor) to the anus, controlling urinary and bowel functions.

Squeezing the PC muscles while holding your breath strongly drives prana from the lower energy centers (Chakras) to the higher energy centers. It is very powerful. Do not hold the breath for longer than 5 seconds.

Repeat the exercise 5 times, taking some time between each exercise to normalize your breathing. After having completed the exercise 5 times, leisurely walk around some 10 to 12 steps before starting the next set of exercises.

The Sunrise Breath

Originally known as the inspirational breath. Movements of the arms are added to the breathing and tensing learned in the previous exercise. The exercise gives us better rotation of the upper body. It releases the muscles of the upper body, the scapula (shoulder blade), the sternum (breast bone) and the ribs.
This exercise prevents and reduces slouching of the shoulders.

Sunrise Breath and the Intercostal Muscles

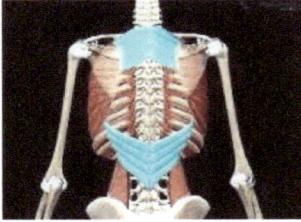

Upper

Action: Elevation of robs# 2 – 5 at the sternocostal and costo vertebrae joints

Innervation: Intercostal nerves.

Arterial supply: Dorsal branches of the superior intercostal arteries

Just in case you may not know:
Dorsal means near the back.
The Intercostal muscles are the small muscles between the ribs, allowing them to move during breathing.
To innervate means to stimulate a nerve in to action.

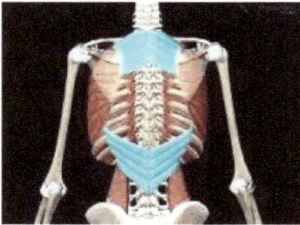

Lower

Action: Depression of ribs 9 – 12 at the sternocostal and costrovertal joints

Innervation: Subcostal nerves

Arterial supply: the dorsal branches pf the inferior intercostal arteries

Sunrise Breath Exercises

- Starting position same as Vital Breath.
- Exhale through the mouth.
- Inhale through the nose, gradually raising your arms palms down on the side to above the head (or as far as is comfortable) with the back of the hands touching up above your head.
- Complete the inhale with a sniff in through the nose and hold.
- Tense your neck muscles, jaws, arms and legs, torso and buttocks, and squeeze your PC muscles.
- Hold to the count of 5.
- Start the exhale by bringing the arms down in four intervals, at 2, 3, 4 and 6 o'clock positions.
- At each interval exhale a portion of air through your teeth.
- Complete the exhale at 6 o'clock with a snort.
- Hold to the count of 5.
- Release all tension.
- Do a couple of normal breaths and pay attention to how your body feels.

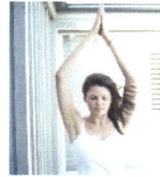

Repeat the exercise 5 times, taking some time between each exercise to normalize your breathing. After having completed the exercise 5 times, leisurely walk around some 10 to 12 steps before starting the next set of exercises.

The Power Breath

Originally known as the perfection breath. A different set of arm movements is introduced and the breathing and tensing is continued.

It releases tension in the torso by easing the erector spinal group of muscles of the trunk, i.e. the Iliocostalis, the longissimus and the spinalis. **The immediate outcome of this exercise is prevention and reduction of upper-back pain.**

Muscles of the Spine

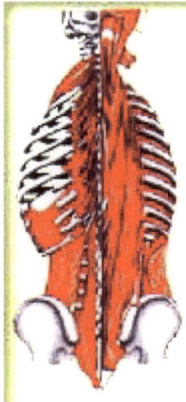

Actions: Extension of the trunk , neck and head at the spinal joints. Lateral flexion of the trunk, neck and head at the spinal joints

Innervation: Spinal nerves

Arterial Supply: The dorsal branches of the posterial innercostal and lumbar arteries

Power Breath Exercises

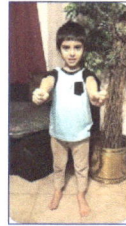

- The starting position is the same as in the Vital Breath.

- Exhale through the mouth.
- During the Inhale gradually bring both arms up, to the front at shoulder height and form fists.
- Complete the inhale with a sniff through the nose and hold.
- Tighten neck, jaws, arms and legs, torso and buttocks and squeeze the PC muscles.
- During the hold swing the arms out to the side and back to front 3 times.
- Continue holding your breath and keep your muscles tight.
- On the exhale bring arms back to the starting position.
- Un-clench your fists and hold to the count of 5.
- Ease all muscles and snort out.
- Do a couple of normal breaths and be aware of how your body feels.

Repeat the exercise 5 times, taking some time between each exercise to normalize your breathing. After having completed the exercise 5 times, leisurely walk around some 10 to 12 steps before starting the next set of exercises.

The Butterfly Breath

Originally known as the perfection breath. The movement is like a butterfly stroke in swimming.

A different set of arm movements is introduced and the breathing and tensing is continued.

It releases tension in the torso by easing the erector spineal group muscles of the trunk, i.e. the Iliocostalis, the longissimus and the spinalis.

The original exercise advised one to keep the arms straight, locked at the elbows which places more strain on the shoulders. I recommend to keep the arms relaxed.

The exercise opens up the ribcage and the diaphragm. It releases tension in the trunk.

It eases muscles that connect to the lumbar plexus.

This exercise in general strengthens the entire back.

The transverso spinalis group are the semispinalis and the multifidus.
The rotators: the Quadrates lumborum, Pectoralis major and minor rectus abdominus.

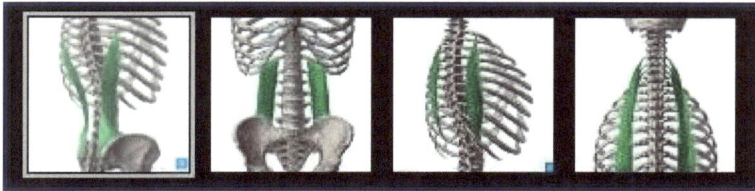

Actions: Extension of the neck, trunk and trunk and the spinal joints
Lateral flexion of the neck, head and spinal joints
Contralateral rotation of the trunk, neck and spinal joints
Anterior tilt of the pelvis at the lumbosacral joint
Ipsolateral rotation of the pelvis and the lumbosacral joint
Innervation: Spinal nerves
Arterior Supply: the occipital artery and the dorsal branches of posterial intercostal and lumber arteries.

Butterfly Breath Exercises

- The starting position is the same as in the Vital Breath.
- Exhale through the mouth.
- During the inhale swing your arms upward and forward, palms facing inward to the eleven o'clock position.

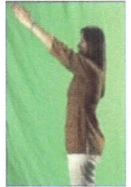

- Complete the inhale with a sniff through the nose, hold and total tense.
- Now swing the arms down and backwards over the head, as close to a perfect circle as you comfortably can, 3 times.
- Exhale until the lungs are empty while bringing the arms down to the side and snort.
- Hold to the count of 5.
- Ease all muscles.
- Do a couple of normal breaths and be aware of how your body feels.

Repeat the exercise 5 times, taking some time between each exercise to normalize your breathing. After having completed the exercise 5 times, leisurely walk around some 10 to 12 steps before starting the next set of exercises.

The Double Back Breath

Originally this exercise was known as the cleansing breath. I named it double back because the movement is similar to a back crawl swimming stroke, except swinging both arms simultaneously. The anatomy of the shoulder will allow only the very agile and limber people to make anything near to a perfect circle. If you cannot do so, that's fine. Do take care not to dislocate the shoulder. The original exercise advised to keep the arms straight, locked at the elbows which places more strain on the shoulders. I recommend to keep the elbows relaxed and slightly bent.

The exercise opens up the energy flow in the pelvis, sacrum and tailbone. It will strengthen the muscles of the pelvis, the psoas major, Iliacus and the psoas minor. **It releases tension in the lower back area, and increases flexibility.**

Double Back Breath and the Lower Back Muscles

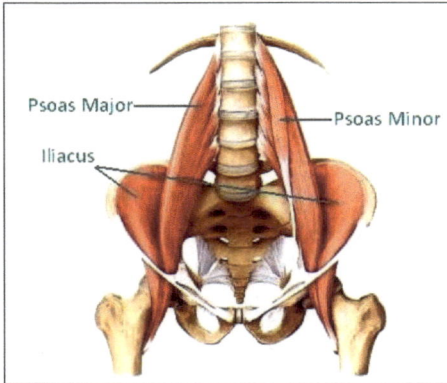

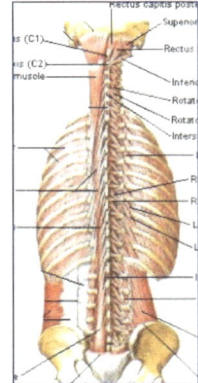

The Psoas Major, Iliacus and Psoas Minor

Action: Flexion of the thigh at the hip joint
Lateral rotation at the hip joint
Flexion of the trunk at the spinal joints
Anterior tilt of the pelvis at the hip joint
Contralateral rotation of the trunk at the spinal joints
Contralateral rotation of the pelvis at the spinal joints
Innervation: Lumbar plexus
Arterial Supply: The lumbar arteries

Double Back Breath Exercises

- The starting position is the same as in the Vital Breath.
- Exhale through the mouth.
- Place your hands on top of each other palms outwards on the tailbone.
- During the inhale swing your arms upward and forward, palms facing inward to the 11 o'clock position.
- Complete the inhale with a sniff. through the nose and hold and tighten.
- During the hold and tense swing the arms over the head and backwards, as close to a perfect circle as you comfortably can.
- Bring arms back to the 'forward and upward' position.
- Do this 2 more times while continuing to hold your breath and keep your muscles tight.
- Exhale till the lungs are empty, snort and bring the arms back to the starting position.
- Hold to the count of 5.
- Ease all muscles.

- Do a couple of normal breaths and be aware of how your body feels.

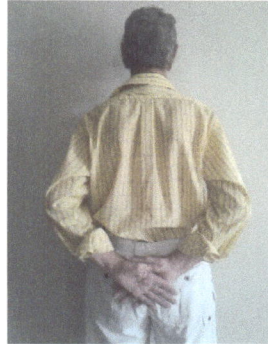

Repeat the exercise 5 times, taking some time between each exercise to normalize your breathing. After having completed the exercise 5 times, leisurely walk around some 10 to 12 steps before starting the next set of exercises.

A story about coming to the Breathing workshop.

My husband told me quite honestly he came with me because he was slightly curious about breathing for good health. Don't we all breathe all the time? What really is energy healing all about?

Climbing the approximately 150 meter, rather steep driveway from the gate to the pool deck, was a challenge the day he came. He had little choice. Few taxi drivers will take their cars to the top. Like me, at the end of his 10 day stay, my husband hiked the driveway without a second thought. The Akimbo Breath was a great challenge, and at the end of the workshop it was no trouble at all.

Those were only two of the changes he told about. After the outing to Rincon de la Vieja, a nearby National Park, he said: "I felt I was able to actually do some hiking. I could not have done these trails before practicing the breathing exercises." He goes on to say: "I am able to think more clearly, I am more agile, more aware, more self-confident. The 10 days of breathing exercises, the walking, and hiking, clean air and (almost) vegetarian diet, drinking water instead of coke have made positive changes in my life. I am healthier and feel better than before I came."

The Akimbo Breath

Originally known as the grand rejuvenation breath. Akimbo is a very Canadian word, referring to the stance with hands on hips taken by Canadian women when chatting to a neighbor across the backyard fence. It may well be the most challenging of the series of exercises. Doing it releases tension of the pelvis and hip area. It eases and strengthens the muscles of the lower back and the buttocks, the gluteus maximus, gluteus medius and gluteus minimus. **Also it prevents, minimizes and corrects the need for adult diapers.**

The Gluteus Muscles

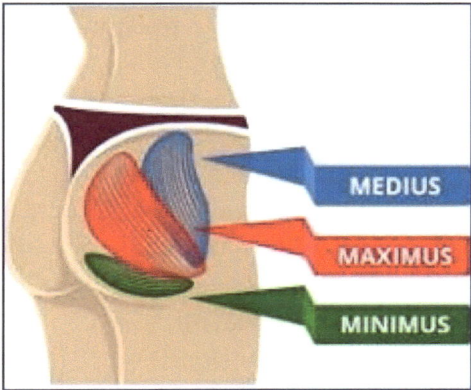

Depression of the pelvis at the hip joint during walking is actually the most important action of the gluteus medius.

Akimbo Breath Exercises

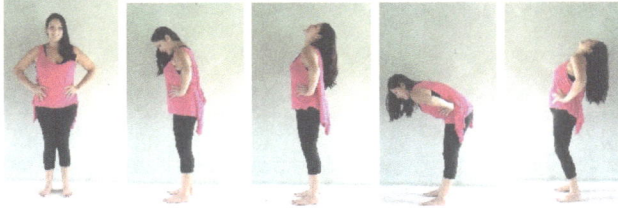

- The starting position is the same as in the Vital Breath.
- Exhale through the mouth.
- Place your hands on your hips as shown with some pressure on the finger tips.
- Inhale, completing with a **sniff** through the nose and hold.
- Tighten.
- Now pivot your head forward until your chin rests on your chest, then tilt back just comfortably, (**bob**) 3 times.
- Bring your head back to upright and exhale, snort and hold, **maintaining the tightness**.
- Without inhaling, **bend** forwards from the hips until your upper body is perpendicular to the floor, then come back and bend back as far as is comfortable, 3 times. Keep your muscles tight.
- Inhale while returning to upright position, sniff.
- Hold to the count of 5 then release all tensions.
- Do a couple of normal breaths and be aware of how your body feels.

Repeat the exercise 5 times, taking some time between each exercise to normalize your breathing. After having completed the exercise 5 times, leisurely walk around some 10 to 12 steps before starting the next set of exercises.

The Charley Chaplin Breath

Originally the exercise was known as the spiritual breath. The movements are reminiscent of the typical Charley Chaplin walking gait.

It releases tension of the pelvis and hip area. The muscles that get the practice are the Pirifirmis Muscle, and the Quadratus Femus Muscle, as well as the Gluteus Muscle. **This exercise helps maintain one's sense of balance.**

For me personally this exercise helped my hearing issues. When doing the exercises in our back yard in Ontario, which is on a hill and the ground is slanted, I initially had a hard time keeping my balance. It gradually improved and a few months later I could stand perfectly balanced while doing this exercise. During the first months my ears continually made popping sounds. Now not so much anymore.

The Piriformis Muscle and Quadratus Femur muscle

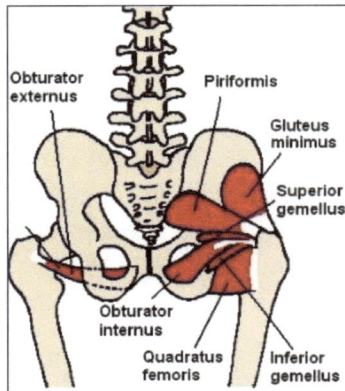

Action: Lateral rotation of the thigh at the hip Joint.
Abduction of the thigh at the hip joint if the thigh is flexed.
Medial rotation of the thigh if the thigh is flexed.
Contralateral rotation at the pelvis at the hip joint
Innervation: Nerve to piriformis and quadratus of the
lumbar-sacral plexus
Arterial Supply: The superior and inferior gluteal arteries

The Charley Chaplin Breath Exercises

- The starting position is the same as in the Vital Breath.
- Exhale through the mouth.
- Place your hands on your hips as shown.
- Inhale through the nose, sniff and hold.
- Tighten.

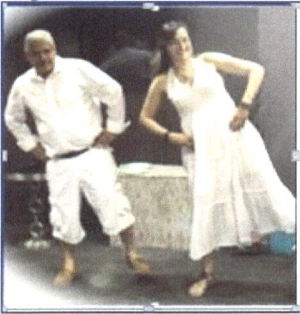

- Lean over to the left as far as you can comfortably until your left heel lifts from the ground.
- Reverse the movement to the right.
- Perform these movements 3 times.
- Return to the starting position, exhale and snort.
- Hold to the count of 5, then release all muscles.
- Do a couple of normal breaths and be aware of how your body feels.

Repeat the exercise 5 times, taking some time between each exercise to normalize your breathing. After having completed the exercise 5 times, leisurely walk around some 10 to 12 steps before starting the next set of exercises.

Now that you are finished with the exercises, simply walk around a bit and resume your daily activities.

DAILY ROUTINE FOR OPTIMUM HEALTH

Start your day with

7 cycles of double nostril breathing.
Do a self-check to see if you are practicing abdominal
breathing.
Confirm your commitment to practice and maintain good
breathing habits.
Spend 5 minutes practicing different breathing rhythms.

At a convenient time

practice an hour of Mentalphysics breathing exercises.

SOURCES

Edwin Dingle
http://www.mentalphysics.net/testimonials/

The Buteyko Method https://en.wikipedia.org/wiki/Buteyko_method

Dr. Andrew Weil
http://www.drweil.com/

Breathing methods.
www.morethanmedication.ca

Dr. Stephen Co
http://pranichealing.com/master-stephen-co

Johnathan Meyers, MD
http://link.springer.com/book/10.1007%2F978-0-387-75246-4

Blood carries oxygen to cells and tissues to support their metabolic activities. Low blood oxygen levels -- also known as hypoxemia -- occur when the level of oxygen in arterial vessels is lower than 80 millimeters of mercury, written as mm Hg. If the oxygen level in the blood is too low, organs like the brain and heart can become hypoxic, meaning they are not receiving enough oxygen to function normally.

The most common effects of low blood and tissue oxygen levels are related to the respiratory system. As such, shortness of breath is generally one of the first symptoms. Anxiety or restlessness, fatigue and headaches are other common symptoms.

Your body needs oxygen to produce the energy needed to function normally. The oxygen you breathe in goes through tiny air sacs in your lungs and into the blood stream, where red blood cells pick it up and carry it throughout the body. **This system can be affected by poor air intake**, poor blood flow or the poor carrying capacity of the red blood cells, leading to low levels of oxygen in the blood.

The book of Common Surgical Diseases, 2008

Author's Note

The information in this booklet provides an overview of the Come Breathe With Us workshop offered by IEHealers. Reading the booklet alone may not provide sufficient practice to master the techniques described. We invite you to contact us to come to a live workshop, when offered at a time and location that is convenient for you to attend.

All of our workshops reflect our intermodal approach to energy healing. The focus of a workshop may well be on one particular modality and the techniques it uses. However, whenever possible, I refer to similar techniques used in other modalities addressing similar issues with the same intent and outcomes. Information about our workshops may be found at www.IEHealers.com

ABOUT THE AUTHOR

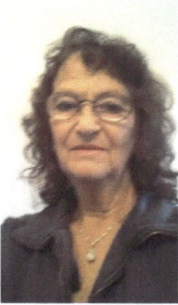

Trudy is an Energy Healing practitioner and instructor. Her experience with hands-on healing reaches back to her childhood. As a child she imitated her mother's healing techniques. She worked with her pet dog and other animals to heal them. In her extended family there were aunts and uncles who also were skilled healers. Other healing modalities she practices include Quantum Touch, Reiki, Psych-K, The Emotion Codes and Dowsing.

Trudy is an experienced and dynamic leader. She engages her audience to participate and enhance their learning experience. Attend a workshop and you can personally experience the positive outcomes of energy healing: rejuvenation, anti-aging, and an opportunity to learn self-healing and healing others. She and her husband Everett live in Newmarket, Ontario during the summer months and in Costa Rica in the winter.

About IEHealers

Our healing journey began at the Oak **&** River Retreat. We have moved onward yet we take the energy of the oak and the river to wherever we go. Our primary focus is wellness orientation, with an emphasis on active personal participation. We are the facilitators - you do the healing. We are rooted in the age-old wisdom of **Hippocrates**: **"The natural healing force within each one of us is the greatest force in getting well"**.

The name of our first Retreat was based on a 300-year-old oak tree that overlooks the property and the river that flows by it. The Oak and the River each on their own and in combination emit energy that transcends time and space.

The Oak embodies strength and empowerment. The flow of the river and the sound of the water rippling over the rocks reverberates fluidity and flexibility, allowing for a free flow of energetic potential.
There remains a place deep within our hearts where we can go, relax, and soak up the peace, the quiet and the power.

No Limits

Most people experience some partial relief as a result of the techniques we practice. However, the healing process is highly individualistic and results vary a great deal from person to person, even for treatment of the same conditions. To quote Alain Herriott:

"I don't know if this [referring to a medical condition] is possible to heal, but I am willing to see what will happen."

Not for Profit

Our business structure is a not for profit sole proprietorship. The facilitators are remunerated according to the Health Industry norm.

We offer an affordable and competitive sliding fee schedule. At the end of each fiscal year, any surplus moneys are deposited into a Trust Fund, which is used to subsidize those for whom the fee structure is not economically feasible.

Disclaimer

In all the work we do, Healing Circles, Workshops, Treatments, Retreats, Distant Healing, we do our utmost to use the healing techniques to the best of our abilities. We offer no guarantees. We can only assure you that we do our best to share what we have to offer. The rest is up to you. Although each of the healing modalities we use is highly effective in promoting maximum health and healing through alternative holistic means, it may not be sufficient intervention for some health-related issues or concerns. Because our treatments may accelerate healing, if you are on medication, we recommend you work closely with your physician to monitor your need for medications, with the intent to reduce your dependency on them. Information contained in our website, through our e-mails, and by phone is not given or intended to be a substitute or replacement for qualified medical advice, diagnosis, or treatment. The owners and facilitators at IEHealers are not engaged in rendering professional or medical advice.

Please take responsibility for your own health!

The Instructors at IEHealers

Everett and Trudy Baker are the founding Quantum-Healing practitioners of IEHealers. We were joined by several other healers over the years. In July 2015 by Miriam Orta, who became qualified to teach Come Breathe With Us. We each have our individual strengths and jointly we work as an amazing team. The energy we run increases exponentially when working together as a team. Individual bios are posted on the website at http://www.IEHealers.com

Other books in the
How Healing Happens Series

Workshops in Energy Healing
Intermodal Energy Healing

These very valuable breathing exercises truly do
improve the body's ability to release stress and to heal.
As with anything that is so simply "good for you",
the easy path is to dismiss something so simple
as a breathing technique as being unimportant.

Jo Lyn Cornelson

www.ingramcontent.com/pod-product-compliance
Lightning Source LLC
Chambersburg PA
CBHW042124290326
41934CB00004BA/185